PANDEMIC
MY STORY

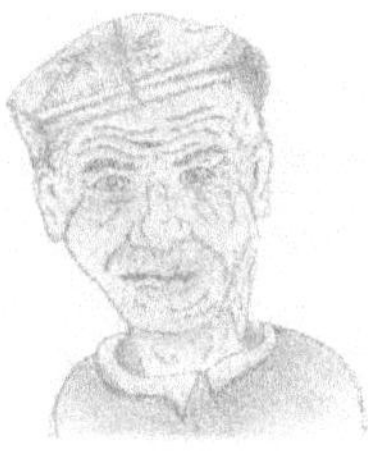

By Scott Dixon

www.thegrumpygit.com

Copyright © Scott Dixon, 2020

ACKNOWLEDGEMENTS

I would like to give credit and thanks to my niece Erin Siddoway for kindly providing me with the design cover for the first edition of my consumer book, the logo for the second edition and subsequent bespoke books.

I would also like to give my heartfelt thanks and gratitude to the nurses, Doctors and NHS staff for their kindness, support, compassion and the treatment I received at the Edinburgh Royal Infirmary hospital.

It takes a special kind of individual to do the job that they are faced with, and I have the utmost respect and admiration for how they handle what they are faced with every day.

I couldn't fault the way I was treated and they saved my life, which I will forever be grateful for.

I would also like to thank friends and family who encouraged me to dial 999 when I was seriously ill and deteriorating fast, as I doubt I would be here to tell the tale now.

Finally, I would like to thank my neighbours and in particular Hannah who kindly fetched my groceries and medication when I was self-isolating and recovering after my hospital admission. Her presence throughout this was clearly meant to be, which I explain further in this book.

CONTENTS

INTRODUCTION

The coronavirus pandemic struck the UK with a vengeance in March 2020 and whilst everyone was aware of it sweeping through Europe with catastrophic results, nobody was prepared for the impact it would have on life as we know it in the UK.

I developed flu-like symptoms on 17th March, which was 6 days before Boris Johnson, the UK Prime Minister, announced a lockdown that would change our lives forever.

This has had a profound impact on everyone's lives, least of all for those who have succumbed to this evil and highly contagious virus.

There is no cure for coronavirus. The symptoms and virus itself are random and unpredictable. All you are given in hospital is Amoxicillin, paracetamols, oxygen and water. Whether you survive or not simply depends on how your immune system reacts to it.

This is my story which takes you from the initial symptoms to being hospitalised and a haphazard recovery which may take years to fully complete.

It has been a harrowing experience that will never leave me and one that I feel compelled to share.

I hope you find this an interesting and engaging read.

WEEK 1 – WHERE IT ALL BEGAN

My life leading up to the first symptoms was as normal as anyone else's. I was fit, healthy and active with no underlying health issues and I would regularly walk up to 8 miles a day around Edinburgh.

I live about 2 miles South of Edinburgh city centre and I could easily walk to Edinburgh Castle or Princes Street in 30 minutes. It's what I would class as an easy walk and one that I regularly enjoyed. It would take up to 20 minutes on the bus for the same journey so it just made sense to me to walk in, get the exercise and fresh air, keep active and my weight in check.

My first symptoms began with an itchy rash on my right wrist. Whilst there is no definitive sign that any particular symptom indicates that you have coronavirus, this is a fairly common one although I didn't know it at the time. I didn't feel or notice anything else that would cause any concerns and this was before anyone had heard of social-distancing and what became commonplace less than 2 weeks later.

I didn't know or realise that I was actively carrying the virus, yet prior to that I was meeting and greeting folk with handshakes, enjoying drinks with a friend in a popular West End bar and doing what we all did without a second thought.

It only lasted for about 48 hours at most, and broke out in to what felt like the start of a cold the following day.

I was able to get showered and ready to attend a 9am appointment the following day. I recall saying that I had the start of a cold coming on, it wasn't anything to worry about and jokingly dismissed it by saying that I didn't have this coronavirus bug that is doing the rounds.

It was just starting to make serious headlines at that point and employers were actively making arrangements for staff to work from home and engage with clients remotely.

I had a wander around the city centre afterwards and popped in to Poundland on Princes Street. I caught sight of the paracetamols and hesitated, wondering if it was worth buying any as I wasn't sure how many I had at home. I put 3 packets in my basket even though I didn't think or feel as though I needed them, strolled around the shop, queued for the self-service checkouts and hopped on and off a couple of buses along Princes Street and through the Southside of Edinburgh to get home.

I wasn't feeling well at this point and took to my bed for the afternoon as I was feeling a bit washed out. I thought it was just the start of a heavy cold, not realising that it would turn in to something much more serious.

COVID-19 was beginning to feature heavily on the news and was coming to the fore in everyone's minds. I don't think that many people really thought it was something to worry too much about at that point as it hadn't really got a grip in the UK, and I thought it was just another version of the flu. I even said that to one of my neighbours and just dismissed it as such.

I woke up the following day and felt as though I had been hit by a sledgehammer. I was able to get up out of bed, showered and do what I had to do but I was really washed out with the symptoms of a heavy cold. I also developed an excruciating headache across the top of my head later that day which was disabling. I took some paracetamols washed down with a glass of water and took to my bed to try and sleep it off.

I couldn't shift this headache at all and I couldn't move from my bed. I had lost my appetite and I was going from bad to worse, spending up to 20 hours a day in bed. I didn't have the energy to get up and cook or even get a glass of water. I was periodically taking paracetamols, Alka Seltzers, Ibuprofen and Co-Codamol to try and shift this debilitating headache to no avail.

My sleeping patterns became haywire and all I could do was just lie in bed and hope that it would pass. I couldn't even get up from my bed to answer the (landline) phone in my lounge. I was becoming breathless with various aches and pains and a fever each morning.

I rang my Doctor's surgery a couple of days later, left a message with the receptionist and my GP returned my call later that morning. I explained my symptoms, answered a few questions and my GP thought it was a viral infection and told me to rest, drink plenty of water and take paracetamols to ease the symptoms. I asked if antibiotics would help and she said that it wouldn't as they are only effective for bacterial infections.

I found a card the following day on my doormat from my new neighbour upstairs. It read;

"Dear Scott,

I hope you are well in these times of 'social-distancing' and fear of being ill! Just to let you know I am still fine and also allowed to work. So if you get affected and need anything, my phone number is: xxx just in case.

Stay well and healthy!

Hannah

PS: I have organised some phone numbers and people in Edinburgh in case I get ill, so don't worry about me!"

She didn't know that I was ill at this point, so it was quite telling that she took the time to reach out to me.

I was beginning to become worried as this just didn't feel like any ordinary cold. I rang 111 that Sunday night and sat on hold for 51 minutes before giving up. My mobile phone package only allows for a 1-hour call before you start getting charged outside your allowance, hence why I chose to hang up.

I had developed a hacking, dry cough and I couldn't stop coughing day and night.

WEEK 2

I was steadily deteriorating and I simply couldn't move with this unbearable and excruciating headache. I was incapacitated and spending up to 20 hours a day in bed. Even getting up to go to the kitchen to get a glass of water would sap me with a sweat followed by diarrhoea.

I would get up at about 6pm to watch some TV and try and have something to eat. I could only cook the simplest of meals and I was having a glass of Guinness most nights to try and keep my iron levels up.

I rang my GP again on Wednesday morning and explained that I had been in touch the week before and how ill I felt. I answered various questions, described my symptoms and yet again it was dismissed as a viral infection with no indication that I may have COVID-19.

I hadn't left the flat for over a week at that point, so for all intents and purposes I was in to my second week of self-isolation.

I was starting to run low on food, although I wasn't really bothered as I couldn't eat much anyway. I had some home-made chicken soup defrosted from the freezer that night with a banana. I had no desire to eat anything, yet I knew that I had to try and do so.

I had lost my sense of taste and smell by the middle of the week and I couldn't taste the Guinness at all that night. It just tasted tinny and I didn't have any desire to finish it, although I did thinking that it would help me.

I swallowed a couple of paracetamols and took a glass of water to bed at 9.30pm that night, only to have to make a sprint to the bathroom and promptly threw up. I couldn't even keep down some chicken soup, water or any tablets.

I had a fairly restful night's sleep that night. I got up at 11am or so to get some home-made soup from the freezer. I couldn't stop coughing, which led to diarrhoea, a temperature and cold sweats.

Friends were convinced that I had coronavirus.

I was deteriorating fast. The cycle of lying in bed awake all hours with a disabling headache and drifting off to sleep each morning, only to wake up with hot and cold sweats became a serious worry. I had no energy at all and I couldn't even have a shower. I was coughing day and night and I had never felt so ill. This was beginning to feel more than a heavy cold or flu.

I rang 111 again that Friday evening and was kept on hold for 40 minutes before giving up, knowing that it was pointless and a waste of time even trying. Family and friends were also becoming worried and my Mother rang that evening. She asked if I thought I had coronavirus and I said that I was convinced at that point that I had it.

It had crossed my mind to dial 999 as a last resort and they all urged me to do so, given how ill I was.

I rang 999 for an ambulance and explained that I could no longer look after myself and I was simply ill. I packed a bag with some clothes, a phone charger and some toiletries. I couldn't think straight at that point and it was simply a last-minute job to throw what I thought I needed, not appreciating or realising that I may end up in hospital for any length of time.

I texted my neighbour upstairs to let her know and said that I would pop my keys through her door.

The ambulance soon arrived and I felt an overwhelming sense of sorrow as I looked around my flat, locked up and slowly walked to the waiting ambulance. This was the first time in my life that I had to request emergency assistance, and living alone not being able to look after yourself at the age of 49 was overwhelming.

I slowly walked down the path at the side of my flat, popped my flat keys through my upstairs neighbour's door and walked to the waiting ambulance. I was asked various questions and my blood pressure, heart rate and oxygen levels were measured and tested.

On the face of it, I was happily able to hold a conversation and probably didn't look ill. In reality, I was and this was my last resort. My GPs had misdiagnosed my symptoms twice, I couldn't get through to 111 and if I hadn't rung 999, I could have died in my bed. That is no exaggeration.

We engaged in a bit of chit-chat and one of them asked if I had problems with my eyes. I was squinting, although I put this down to the fact that I had been confined to my bed in a dark room for up to 20 hours a day for almost 2 weeks and I was sat in a brightly lit environment with high intensity LED lights.

My blood pressure and oxygen levels were slightly low and the upshot of it was that they didn't think that I was ill enough to warrant a trip to hospital. I was in despair at that point and had to plead with them that I could no longer look after myself. I couldn't find the energy to have a shower or leave my bed to answer the phone in the lounge, so the thought of having to return to my flat to deal with this was impossible for me to comprehend.

They both agreed to take me to the hospital and some paperwork had to be prepared and completed in advance for the handover at A & E. This took a few minutes and I was strapped in to my seat with a seatbelt whilst one of the paramedics sat by me for the 2-mile journey to the Edinburgh Royal Infirmary. The roads were deserted apart from a Police car sat near a usually busy roundabout by a nearby shopping centre.

The ambulance pulled up at the A & E red zone which was set aside for those who are admitted with suspected COVID-19 symptoms. A member of staff was waiting with a wheelchair for me and I was swiftly taken in to testing area and asked to lie on a bed with the backrest tilted at a 45-degree angle.

It quickly became apparent that I was dehydrated and I was put on an intravenous drip to have a litre of fluids pumped in to my body. Various tests were taken including a blood test followed by a chest x-ray. The blood test showed lymphopenia and a CRP (C-Reactive Protein) level of over 200 which was considered dangerous with inflammation. The chest x-ray results finally concluded that I had patches of pneumonia on my lungs and this triggered a COVID-19 test.

COVID-19 tests are only taken if you are going to be admitted to hospital to all incoming patients. If you are considered well enough to go home, you are not given the chance to have a test even though you may be a carrier of the disease.

The test involves having a swab taken from the back of your throat and up your nostrils. I was warned that it may make me gag, although it didn't and it wasn't uncomfortable. Hardly pleasant, although these things never are!

I was then wheeled away on the same bed to an isolation ward with one other patient across from me. I had a quiet night's sleep and rest, which was only interrupted by oxygen and heart rate tests every 2 hours. This was to be the only quiet night's sleep and rest that I was going to get during my stay in hospital.

I woke up the following morning and had some cereal and coffee. The nurse gave me the start of a course of Amoxicillin, paracetamols and a jug of iced water. I just lay there wiped out and feeling ill and nauseous.

I couldn't walk across the ward to the bathroom without feeling somewhat dizzy, unsteady on my feet and feeling nauseous. I explained that to one of the nurses shortly afterwards and she gave me some tablets which alleviated it fairly quickly. My oxygen levels were tested and found to be slightly below normal so I was put on oxygen to remedy it.

I passed the time browsing social media and the Internet on my phone before engaging in a bit of chat with a young lad who was admitted for epilepsy and seizures the previous day. We were both in isolation on the same ward, yet he showed no signs of having COVID-19 and was in the same proximity with me who was. He was tested on admission as everyone is, yet was kept in isolation with me and had to use a shared bathroom that was not cleaned or disinfected in that time.

I didn't think anything of it at the time as we were both waiting on our results. He was also waiting for a consultation with a Doctor based on various epilepsy tests.

The Doctor came in late that morning to speak to him and he was told that his COVID-19 test was negative. He had the option to leave immediately or wait until 9pm and be kept under observation as a precaution. He chose the latter and it was originally mooted that he would be taken to a general ward.

He didn't seem too concerned and he passed the time having video conference calls with family and friends.

A reality check soon came shortly afterwards when he asked if he could pop to the shop. That was the point when he was told that the decision had been reversed and he couldn't leave the ward until my results came through. He had no choice now and was relying on my results.

I was too poorly to engage in much chit-chat at all and a fairly quiet and uneventful few hours passed.

My Doctor came on to the ward at 3.45pm to see me. I remember the time and moment vividly. He engaged in a few moments of general conversation and asked how I was feeling before breaking the news to me that I had been tested positive for COVID-19. It struck me like a lightning bolt. I saw it coming in a way, I was somehow expecting it yet nothing can prepare you for the moment that you are told that you have an incurable disease. I sat agog and the first thoughts that came to mind were, *"Am I going to die?"* The Doctor didn't seem too concerned at all and conveyed the impression that I didn't have much to worry about, but that did not allay my initial thoughts.

The Doctor left the ward moments later and the young lad sat across from me was in a state of shock. He said, *"Sorry to hear that mate".* I didn't really have time to give a reply as I quickly rang my parents to let them know before a couple of nurses swiftly came in to get me to another ward as quickly as possible.

I will never know what his outcome was. He was tested negative hours earlier, yet he may have contracted it from me in the time that we were on that ward from the bathroom that we both used which was never cleaned or disinfected.

Moments later I found myself on a different ward with 3 elderly gentleman all over the age of 70. One across from me didn't appear to be too ill at all and was more able and mobile than me, whilst the other two were in a bad way. One gentleman next to me was bed-ridden with a catheter fitted that he thought wasn't working properly, which seemed to make him more agitated than any other ailments that he had.

The bed space across from me appeared to be on rotation for seriously ill patients that required oxygen masks and were confined to their beds. It appeared to be a holding space if you were borderline needing admission to the Intensive Care Unit while they continually assessed the condition of the patient.

I just lay there with only my phone to keep me occupied. The day was broken up by regular visits from the nurses to check oxygen levels and blood pressure, administer medication and meals.

My neighbour kindly texted me whilst I was in hospital asking how I was and said,

"Just let me know what you need. I am working from home and in good health (for now). I have my bike so I won't need to go on the bus! You were really fortunate there! Well, if you get home, you will need to isolate until you are better, and then you are probably immune (with such strong inflammatory response, you must have loads of antivirus antibodies!), so you will be able to go everywhere you want without being afraid! They may even ask you to donate your

blood to help other patients. But first get better! Hope they let you rest now".

I really appreciated her text and the offer of help. It was very comforting at a time when there was in all honesty little comfort to be found.

The hospital menu choices really surprised me and the quality of the food was exemplary. I enjoyed the best home-made minestrone and tomato soup and the roast chicken dinner was hearty and tasty. It's fair to say that helped in my recovery as prior to that I had lost my appetite and I had hardly eaten much at all for about a week. I had lost 9lb in as many days before my hospital admission.

Both of these gentlemen swallowed up so much time between about 6 nurses day and night. The gentleman next to me became more agitated and irascible as the weekend progressed, which was exacerbated as night fell and the lights were dimmed.

Everything is magnified in the hours of darkness on a hospital ward. It was a Saturday night and there was a skeleton staff on duty when the first of two power outages took place at around midnight. It may have been a test for the back-up generators or a power cut. Nobody knew, but it set this gentleman off and he began protesting loudly. He was deaf when it suited him so anything said by me, the gentleman opposite or the nurses literally fell on deaf ears.

The nurses were running around outside of our ward trying to figure out what was happening, having to fully kit themselves before entering our ward to try and offer an explanation and reset any of the machines.

The same thing happened again about half an hour later and the protests from the gentleman next to me were much louder.

He began complaining loudly that the power cuts were intolerable, he was freezing cold and he was most uncomfortable. He also decided that he wanted his teeth cleaned at 1.15am. The nurse tried to explain that people are trying to sleep and that it's not possible but he wasn't having it. He began repeatedly shouting at the top of his voice, *"I WANT MY TEETH CLEANED"*. He then shouted, *"MY MOUTH IS FOUL. I WANT MY TEETH CLEANED"*. This prompted me to loudly agree with him and saying that his manners were too, although he had selective deafness so it's doubtful he would have heard me.

Everyone on the ward was awake at this point and annoyed by his antics. The only way the nurse could pacify him was to do what he demanded.

The seriously ill gentleman across from me was on oxygen and just couldn't settle. He was continually tossing and turning and calling for assistance. The nurses never stopped that night between the two of them and had to check everyone's oxygen levels and blood pressure every 2 hours as well.

There was no way I was going to get any sleep or rest that night. It was like being in a horror movie. The poor staff who have to deal with this was upsetting to see.

I was drifting on and off throughout the night and pretty much gave up early on Sunday morning. I took to Twitter and wrote, *"My God, the howls of pain on this coronavirus ward will never leave me. It is worse than you can ever imagine. Please adhere to the advice – you really wouldn't want to be where I am right now. It's so difficult to cope with for everyone involved".*

This tweet was liked 180 times, retweeted 52 times and viewed by 36,933 people on Twitter at the time of writing this.

The incident I was referring to happened at 5am that Sunday morning. It was absolute chaos with nurses trying to calm and settle those in so much agony. I just lay in my bed wondering what my life had come to and shed some tears.

I couldn't do anything without it setting off uncontrollable coughing, sweats and panic attacks. I thought I had turned a corner the previous day but I didn't think I would be out as soon as I had hoped. I felt ill as soon as I tried to do anything.

I was touched and moved by the flood of messages that followed on that thread and privately from complete strangers who reached out to me offering their sympathy and support.

They moved the most disruptive and seriously ill patient on to another ward. I could only surmise that he needed ITU treatment, although there was no way of knowing. This appeared to be a rotating bed space that was used for borderline cases where patients were monitored and assessed before being moved on, presumably to ITU.

I was feeling quite overwhelmed and emotional at this point. I was completely exhausted and simply ill.

Incredibly, one of the nurses put a request out on Facebook for toiletries as most COVID-19 patients are admitted in just the clothes they arrived in and nothing else. This prompted a flood of donations from kind-hearted well-wishers and we received over £10,000 worth of gifts. Tesco across the

Lothians donated pyjamas and clothing whilst others donated iPads, toiletries and all sorts of gifts to help those who needed them most.

It's quite emotional even now to think about it and it had me in tears at the time. I didn't have any deodorant, shower gel, razers or shaving foam as I literally just had a few minutes to pack my bag after dialling 999 and I wasn't thinking straight. I hadn't had a shave for about a week or a shower for a few days as I simply didn't have the energy to do so. This really touched me and restored my faith in humanity when I was at my lowest ebb.

Sunday was an uneventful day compared to the night before. The peace was only broken when the nurses had to try and bathe the bed-ridden gentleman next to me that morning. He appeared to have bed sores from being incapacitated with a catheter that he didn't think was working properly, which exacerbated his protests.

The howls and screams of pain could only be compared to that of a scalded cat. I have literally never heard anything like it in my life. The poor nurses were trying to pacify him but there was no way they could. The screams were interspersed with what sounded like a purring noise as they were bathing him, and the nurses asked if he was in pain as they weren't sure. Moments later the screams started again and this would last for up to half an hour each morning.

He had a penchant for hot, sweet tea and would regularly press the buzzer for attention. A nurse would come through and he would ask slowly, *"Can I have some hot, sweet tea?"* That would prompt a follow-up question, *"How would you like it?"*, which was met with, *"I can't hear you?"* I knew how he liked his tea off by heart as this was a regular pantomime so I would chime in with, *"3 sugars, no milk, in a plastic beaker"*.

One thing that shocked and surprised me was the lack of Personal Protective Equipment (PPE). The nurses were only given plastic disposable gloves, a face mask and a plastic apron to wear over their uniforms. These had to be worn and disposed of every time they left the ward. The nurses are putting their lives on the line to do their job and I expected much better protection to be provided.

I don't know how they could be so cheerful, chatty and compassionate under such demanding and stressful circumstances. It was truly admirable and touching to see.

My oxygen levels had improved later that day and I was taken off oxygen at lunchtime. The anti-sickness tablets I was given 24 hours earlier and prescribed once a day had worked wonders and I enjoyed a delicious and hearty roast chicken dinner. My appetite and sense of taste and smell was beginning to return and I had felt as though I had turned a corner, although it was too soon to tell.

I engaged in a bit of chit-chat with the gentleman across from me that afternoon. He had recently returned from a holiday in Benidorm with his wife and they both fell ill with COVID-19 shortly afterwards. He thought that he had caught it out there, although there is no way of knowing. His wife was on a ward next door and the nurses had kindly arranged for him to meet up with her. This lifted his spirits immensely and they took him in a wheelchair so they could spend some time together.

We both shared our love for the resort and swapped anecdotes about various bars, tribute acts and venues around the town. He would go a few times each year, whereas I normally go each Christmas and meet up with a friend from Leeds who does the same. It was a good way to pass the time in the absence of anything else.

Another restless and sleepless night followed on the ward with the pattern being much the same, with two patients demanding constant attention to the detriment of myself and another gentleman who simply wanted to get some sleep.

The bed-ridden gentleman next to me was just giving the nurses the run-around 24/7 and was simply demanding, obnoxious and rude towards the nurses who were trying to do their best for everyone. It was chaotic and stressful to deal with and I was beginning to wonder how I was meant to rest and recover fully. This certainly wasn't the Premier Inn where you are guaranteed a good night's sleep!

WEEK 3

It was Monday morning and one of the nurses came around shortly after 7am to ask for everyone's breakfast requests. I simply asked for cereal and a coffee and the Doctor began their morning visit to speak to each patient individually.

COVID-19 affects everyone in different ways and it is by nature random and unpredictable.

The Doctor came to me and asked how I was feeling? I said that I was tired and there was no way anyone on the ward could get any rest, recuperate and recover properly when we had such a disruptive and rude patient on the ward. I was referring to the bed-ridden irascible gentleman beside me.

His response was to say that I was to be discharged that afternoon as I was considered medically fit and able to go home. I felt ill and I just looked at him in disbelief. The measure used is that if you are able to walk, shower and breathe unaided you are able to go home. I said that I didn't feel well enough to go home and look after myself, which the Doctor countered by saying that I ran a high risk of catching a super-infection in the hospital and that I would recover quicker at home.

I then asked how I was meant to get home and said that I didn't have any family or friends that could collect me. He said that I would just have to get a taxi later in the afternoon instead.

I was gobsmacked at hearing that, knowing that it wasn't beyond the wit of anyone to arrange for a patient transfer for a 2-mile journey. That aside, I considered it wholly unfair and unacceptable to put taxi drivers and anyone else at risk knowing how highly infectious this disease is.

The decision had been made though.

In the meantime, my neighbour (Hannah) texted me asking, *"Do you need anything there? Like toothbrush or clean underwear or so? I will go grocery shopping again, so I can get you something from the stores if you need anything. I think they allow people to 'deliver' a package to the hospital".*

She didn't know that I was coming home later that day. I was conscious that she only had a bicycle to carry my shopping so I just asked her to simply get me 6 medium eggs, a small loaf, bananas and some milk.

She replied with, *"Great! Hope you feel well enough! Sure you don't need anything like soup or something resembling dinner? I'll be going to Sainsburys for my own stuff anyway, so I can get you anything. Do you have medicines like paracetamol as well?"*

I replied by saying, *"I am fine for everything else thanks Hannah. No idea on times so tomorrow will be fine…appreciate it. This ward is a nightmare".*

We are lucky where we both live as Cameron Toll Shopping Centre is literally half a mile away and has virtually everything you need including stores such as Aldi, Boots, Sainsburys, Greggs, Poundland and various other stores that most outlets have nowadays.

I knew that I had enough provisions to get me through another 2 weeks of self-isolation and I just needed the basics.

Most people who live in a city tend to just pick up groceries 'as and when' whilst you're out and about as we are spoilt for choice with every shop you can think of mostly within walking distance.

I spent the rest of that morning just lying in bed wondering how I was going to cope when I got home. I had spent a fortnight confined to my bed before I was admitted to hospital, yet days later I was considered fit and able to go home and manage my own recovery.

In the meantime, the elderly gentleman next to me was becoming more exasperated and demanding attention from the nurses. He kept shouting, *"I WANT TO DIE. I WANT TO DIE. I HAVE HAD ENOUGH OF THIS",* and complaining how cold and uncomfortable he was. One of the nurses said in a compassionate tone, *"Ahh, don't say that",* and tried to pacify him. This lasted for about half an hour before he drifted off to sleep. Ironically, he would sleep for up to 20 hours a day and would only wake up and create chaos to coincide with the times everyone else was trying to sleep.

I had my lunch and a couple of nurses came round shortly afterwards to say that I had to get ready and pack my bag as they needed to strip the bed. I sat in the chair beside the bed and mentioned to one of the nurses about the travel arrangements (or lack of) that I was faced with and the risks posed to those who are expected to assist.

I was surprised when she said that infected people are wandering around everywhere and I would have a mask. I expected other arrangements to be in place under the circumstances and not left to my own devices to arrange my return home. These were legitimate concerns I had not just for myself but for others, yet it was just dismissed as 'one of those things'. I simply thought it was unfair and unacceptable.

A couple of Edinburgh Researchers came to see me shortly before I was discharged to ask if I would be happy to give some samples to assist with the World Health Organisation (WHO) research study involving people who have recently acquired COVID-19.

The rationale was to enable the research study gain important information about COVID-19 so they can try and find better ways to manage and treat it in future.

I was more than happy to do so and I gave a blood and urine sample together with a swab sample from my mouth, nose and throat.

The researchers left and a nurse came through to the ward moments later with my bag of medication that would last me a fortnight to take home. I was sat in the chair for as long as possible and said that I still felt ill, even though that wasn't going to make any difference at that point. She sympathised, explained what I needed to take and avoid, wished me well and left.

My time to leave came at 3pm and I was called to the reception area by a nurse who said that I was ready to be discharged. I tied my paper mask over my face and shook hands with the elderly gentleman and Benidorm acquaintance who I had built up a rapport with. We both wished each other all the best and said that our paths may cross one day in Benidorm. Stranger things have happened, although we didn't exchange phone numbers or contact details.

I picked up my medication from the reception desk by the ward, thanked the nurses for everything that they did for me and asked for directions to the taxi rank.

I had to walk some distance through the corridors, down in the lift and via more corridors and out towards the taxi rank nearby the main entrance. I was breathless and exhausted. It was in the forefront of my mind that I was carrying an infectious disease and nobody knew, least of all the taxi drivers on duty who are unknowingly carrying discharged patients who are touching doors, seats and handles with no disinfectant on board. The risks this carries to other passengers afterwards is obvious, and this is magnified on public transport.

I was able to get a black cab straight away from the waiting queue of taxis on the rank. The driver was protected by a Perspex screen and I was home within 10 minutes. I was given the option to pay in cash or by card. I chose to pay by card to avoid the risk of transmitting the disease to the driver, as he didn't know that he was carrying a passenger who had coronavirus.

I was home much sooner than I had hoped and expected and in somewhat of a daze with disbelief at it all. I just dropped my bag in the kitchen, threw my paper mask in the kitchen bin and flaked out asleep in bed for about 2 hours. I felt alone, vulnerable and in need of care and support yet here I was discharged to just fend for myself.

I made a couple of phone calls and texted my neighbour upstairs to let her know that I was back home.

I still felt seriously ill, and the Doctor at the hospital said that would be the case for at least another fortnight when I voiced my concerns about how I was meant to look after myself. My appetite was slowly returning at that point after having some hearty and delicious food during my hospital stay, although I didn't have the energy or desire to cook anything. I was simply washed out and gaunt in my appearance. I took a glass of water to my bed and spent up to 16 hours in bed that night.

Hannah, my neighbour, texted me the following morning saying,

"Hope you had a good night. I'll be going for groceries in a minute. When I'm back, I'll put your groceries in front of your door and text you, so you know they are there".

I was feeling breathless and wiped out, although I was well enough to get showered and to make a sandwich.

We kept in touch throughout the week as I was still confined to my bed for up to 16 hours a day. I was only given 7 days of antibiotics and I was worried that I needed some more to complete my recovery.

I rang the Doctor's surgery on Thursday morning and a GP returned my call. This was the third different GP I had spoken to since I began feeling ill. She apologised for what she described as a 'clunky experience', and explained that they are still learning about the virus and the symptoms. She explained that antibiotics are only effective for up to about 10 days and extended my prescription for another 3 days. I asked how I could get my neighbour to collect it for me, and she said that she would fax it through to a pharmacy nearby that could cope with the demand. My neighbour simply needed to give my name and date of birth to collect it.

Hannah, my neighbour, kindly went to the pharmacy to collect my prescription and popped it through my door.

I was still struggling with a persistent cough and shortness of breath, but I was slowly improving as each day passed. I was conscious that she could hear it from her flat above me and I apologised for it, although there was nothing I could do. My lungs felt as though they had been wrecked by this virus and I had aged so much. I had never felt so vulnerable and worried for my wellbeing. I was still spending 12 – 16 hours a day in bed and everything was a struggle. I did wonder how (or even) when I would fully recover from this and hardly a day went by when I didn't shed a few tears in despair.

WEEK 4

This was the first time I was able to get out of bed before 9am. It was the start of a new week and I was trying to get back in to some sort of routine again. I was able to shower daily again and my appetite was slowly returning. I weighed myself and I had lost about 10lb and my weight was 11st 6lb. It was weight that I could afford to lose, although it was a drastic amount and I knew I had to try and build myself up again.

I used to walk up to 40 miles a month around Edinburgh before I fell ill. I could barely walk around my flat without struggling for breath, and even standing in the shower for a few minutes left my legs weak and unsteady. This virus had simply floored me. I knew that I was one of the lucky ones, and I was faced with a haphazard process to recovery. Every day was a struggle and I was at a very low ebb. This virus is brutal and it had broken me.

Every day was much the same, although I was slowly spending less time in bed and able to sit outside in my garden and recuperate in the warm sunshine and fresh air.

WEEK 5

Tuesday morning proved to be a revelation. I tweeted,

"I only found out today my new neighbour is a biologist and popped a note with her contact details through my door if I got ill and needed anything, not realising that I was deteriorating with COVID-19 and was hospitalised days later. So kind and thoughtful – I am fortunate".

Can you imagine finding out that your new neighbour, who only moved in to the flat above you last Christmas, was a biologist and researcher who knew everything about coronavirus and had the foresight to reach out to you in the early stages of the outbreak. The chances of that are remote, and I took that as a sign that she was sent to me as a Guardian Angel to watch out for me in my hour of need.

An elderly neighbour, who is in her 70s and doesn't own a car, actually walked half a mile each way to Aldi and left quite a heavy bag on my doorstep containing bread, eggs, milk, bottles of lager and various other groceries. She simply sent me a text afterwards to say that she had left a bag outside my front door. I was astonished and so appreciative of her kindness, as I hadn't asked her to get me anything and I would never have expected her to do that.

All of the neighbours in our sleepy cul-de-sac knew that I had been admitted to hospital weeks earlier as they saw the ambulance parked outside. We don't see much of each other and mostly pass like ships in the night, so to say that I was surprised is an understatement.

I was finally able to leave my flat that Friday afternoon on 10th April for the first time in about a month to drive again and actually do a food shop. It felt wonderful. I still had a long way to go but this was probably the best day so far.

I drove half a mile to Cameron Toll Shopping Centre, parked up and slowly strolled across the car park to join the fairly short queue of shoppers waiting 2 metres apart in a line to get in to Aldi.

This was the first time I had been out for over a month and the first time since lockdown began on 23rd March. The roads were empty as was the vast car park which surrounds Cameron Toll. Everything felt different and the pace of life felt much slower. I can imagine Christmas Day being like this in Edinburgh, yet this was Good Friday and Easter Bank Holiday weekend.

Good Friday is a normal working day in Scotland in lieu of 2nd January, which is a Bank Holiday for the Scots to recover from the Hogmanay revelry.

One thing I noticed was the significant minority that were not social-distancing in supermarkets. The number of people who came up close to me was unbelievable. I was probably still carrying the virus and I still had somewhat of a persistent cough, yet nobody knew and I couldn't say anything without sparking chaos and uproar. Nobody knows who has the virus or is recovering from it, yet some people think that it won't affect them until it does.

I felt as though I shouldn't be out, yet I didn't really have much choice as I had spent 2 weeks of self-isolation before and after being hospitalised and I badly needed to do a proper food shop. I couldn't get any groceries delivered due to the demand on the delivery slots and there was no way I could register as being vulnerable to jump the queue. The supermarkets in England had access to lists of vulnerable customers, but Scotland was weeks behind in following suit.

I was able to get virtually everything I needed. I bought a 1 litre bottle of flavoured water as I knew that I would need a drink after I had paid for my groceries. I was exhausted and I didn't have the strength to open it, so I had to ask one of the checkout staff to do so for me.

It was great to finally be independent again and not rely on the kindness of my neighbours to get my groceries.

I was lucky with the weather too with endless days of warm sunshine and cool fresh air which lasted for the whole of April.

My back garden gets the sun virtually all day and it was a joy to just sit outside in it. Never underestimate the simple pleasure of being able to sit outside and have your breakfast in the quiet surroundings of your own back garden after being so ill.

Sitting out in the garden each day soaking up the sun was working wonders in clearing up the persistent cough I had and the lingering side-effects of the virus. I was feeling better as each day passed. I also looked much better as my appetite had returned and I was beginning to tan well.

My lawn hadn't been cut since last October and was becoming an eyesore, although I was in no fit state to do anything about it. I would periodically get up from my camping chair to do a bit of weeding, only to have to sit back down again after a few minutes as I was becoming breathless and my legs were so weak.

Chronic fatigue complete with a persistent cough and weak and aching legs was a problem that would prove to be problematic to deal with.

I left an Easter egg outside my neighbour's door on Easter Sunday and texted her to let her know whilst I got a paper, only to find a home-made hot cross bun by mine when I returned. I made a point of driving to Aldi that afternoon to buy her some tulips and apple and cinnamon hot cross buns along with my essentials. It seemed quite appropriate as she is from the Netherlands!

WEEK 6

It's a complicated recovery. Good days followed by bad days. Chronic fatigue, breathing problems, feeling normal energy-wise then having to sit down after a few minutes, vivid and strange dreams.

When my symptoms began on 17th March, I didn't know what to expect. Nobody really knew much about the virus, which may explain why I was missed twice by GPs on telephone consultations. We all now know much more about the virus and symptoms, although we still don't know much about the long-term impact on health, the possibility of immunity, how long infected patients remain contagious or what the recovery looks like.

Those who do not fully rest and recover from COVID-19 risk having Chronic Fatigue Syndrome or ME (Myalgic Encephalomyelitis) for life. That preyed on my mind when I was told that by a journalist on Twitter. My sleeping patterns were all over the place, although I was feeling better as each day passed. I still had a persistent, dry, niggling cough and I wondered how much damage had been done to my lungs as a result of the virus.

The endless fine, warm and sunny weather was working wonders though and I made the most of it by spending hours sat outside to recuperate and try to restore my health as quickly as possible.

My lawn hadn't been cut since last October and was an eyesore, least of all for my neighbour upstairs who had to look at it each day. I finally got it cut and strimmed one morning, which took the best part of 2 hours and spent the rest of the day resting. It was simply too much for me physically and my legs were like jelly and aching for days afterwards.

My appetite had returned and I was beginning to regain the weight I had lost. Coupled with a good tan, I was beginning to look and feel much healthier. The weakness in my legs was an ongoing problem and a worry though. To think that a few weeks earlier I was able to walk up to 8 miles at a time easily, yet a few minutes of weeding at a time was making me breathless and having to sit down and rest despaired me.

Another unusual side-effect of this illness is weird, random and vivid dreams, although many people have echoed the same simply due to the lockdown. Maybe it's boredom, a lack of routine or something else – I don't know. One dream had me hosting a surprise party with Piers Morgan as a relative he had never met and riding around Thailand on a scooter! I'm sure Piers would be delighted to know that!

I have never been to Asia and the Far East, so I don't know where the other dream came from. I did ride and own scooters for over 20 years though. It was a way of life when I lived in the Isle of Man, which was great fun over the years and saw me travel from the Isle of Man up to Shetland and around the North East of England.

The flat next door to me is owned by an elderly lady who is 96-year-old and remains unoccupied as she can no longer look after herself. I did say quite some time ago that I would look after her small garden and that was also becoming an eyesore. I know what it's like to have bad neighbours (as many of us know), and the neighbours upstairs and at the side had to look at this each day. It took me 2 hours to cut, weed and tidy it up one morning. I sat and rested in the sun that afternoon and my legs were as stiff as boards the following day. I suffered for it for days afterwards, and all I could do was rest and do as little physical activity as possible.

Even 10 minutes of vacuuming would result in my back and legs beginning to ache. I suddenly felt old before my time, and there were times when I would sit and shed a few tears thinking and wondering how I was going to overcome this.

It's a double-edged sword though. You need to do some physical activity to build your strength back up, yet you can't do too much because you risk suffering from Chronic Fatigue Syndrome or ME for life. Finding that balance was always going to be tricky.

WEEK 7

The end of April marked a milestone insofar as turning 50-year-old. I recall January 2020 with high hopes and expectations thinking, *"This will be my year",* yet here I was recovering from coronavirus. 2020 was going to be the year when the bins went out more than me!

I am one of the lucky ones, although any sort of light exercise or physical activity would leave my legs aching for days afterwards. I couldn't stand for more than a few minutes without feeling an overwhelming weakness in my legs and needing to sit down. Breathlessness was still a problem, and even having a shower would trigger slight gasping for air. I felt as though I had aged literally overnight.

It was a bright, cool and fairly cloudy day with sunny spells and only 9c, although it was pleasant enough to sit in a sheltered spot by my kitchen door in the sunshine and have my breakfast. I made a couple of phone calls, took part in a Zoom call with fellow bloggers, had some lunch and drove in to the city centre for a gentle stroll around the city.

I have never seen Edinburgh so eerily quiet with deserted streets and closed shops everywhere. I was left wondering how shopkeepers, bars, restaurants, cafes and everything else which largely revolves around tourism would bounce back from this. Everything that I and everyone else had taken for granted was gone at the stroke of a pen.

I had a slow wander through Princes Street Gardens and sat down on one of the memorial benches to rest. The skies were beginning to clear and I was sat overlooking a row of multi-coloured tulips lining a neatly trimmed hedge, well-kept gardens and trees surrounding the bandstand nestled under the granite rock and Castle.

Edinburgh really shines at this time of year with cherry blossom bursting everywhere and over 100 public gardens and plenty of green spaces to enjoy the fresh air.

This isn't quite how I expected to mark my 50th birthday, although it was pleasant enough and I shared it with a friend via a video call.

I was lucky with the weather throughout the whole of April with endless blue skies, warm sunshine and cool air to sit out in. I spent a lot of time simply just soaking it up in the garden and I had a healthy glow. My appetite had fully recovered, I had gained most of the weight that I had lost and I was gradually building my strength back up by doing some light gardening.

I had signed up for the World Health Organisation (WHO) research programme with the researchers at Edinburgh University so they can get a better understanding of how the coronavirus works. I agreed to a follow-up appointment at the Edinburgh Royal Infirmary hospital.

I live only a few minutes' drive away and there was a funeral cortege leaving the hospital for a long-serving nurse who had died of coronavirus. The entrance and surrounding paths were lined with staff and visitors clapping as the hearse and cortege left the hospital. All vehicles stopped as a mark of respect, and it was quite moving to see.

What shocked me as I strolled around the hospital was a complete lack of social-distancing. Everyone was directed to the hand sanitizers at the entrance, yet after that it was pretty much a free for all with nobody adhering to any guidelines whatsoever.

I was tested again for coronavirus complete with blood and urine tests. I was told that if there were any concerns, they would be in touch. No news would literally be good news.

I left the hospital feeling emotional knowing that I wasn't out of the woods yet. It felt like a setback that I wasn't expecting, and I had to yet again do another proper food shop in case I had to self-isolate for the third time.

I came home, unpacked my groceries, had some lunch and flaked out in bed fast asleep all afternoon. Any sort of exercise just left me completely worn out and exhausted.

I was beginning to wonder how long my recovery would take. I still had a bit of a niggling cough; some breathlessness and my legs were still weak and ache if I did much. 10 minutes of vacuum cleaning a few days earlier had left me with an aching back, breathless and aching legs which led to me having to sit down and rest. My legs were the main problem at this point really, and I would have to spend any time sat down with them resting on a foot cushion.

The chronic fatigue, persistent cough and breathlessness were slowly and gradually fading, although it was a process that was hard to measure as it had been so prolonged. I understand that it may take up to 18 months for my lungs to fully recover from the scarring to my lungs from pneumonia. The virus attacks the lungs and I was found to have patches of pneumonia and inflammation, which is the result of the immune system's response to the infection.

I was getting flashbacks from my stay in hospital and it wouldn't take much to trigger tearful emotions since I was discharged from hospital. There is no way of knowing what the long-term physical or mental consequences are, which will vary depending on each individual's experience.

I have had heavy colds and flu in the past but this was very different, and I was left wondering if any permanent damage had been done to my health and immune system. This virus is brutal and attacks your body in a way that nothing else does, and it will probably be never the same again.

The lockdown didn't really bother me as I had no inclination to go far or do much. Like most people, I would have liked to have been able to go for a drive somewhere for a change of scenery but it wasn't a priority. I was more focused on trying to restore my health and gradually building up my strength by doing some light gardening and chores at home.

WEEK 8

I was waiting for a phone call from the hospital, which never arrived and signalled that all was well and there were no further concerns from the recent follow-up tests.

I felt well and able enough to leave the flat for the first time in 2 months on foot and go for a decent walk. I live 2 miles from Edinburgh Castle, which I would normally be able to cover in 30 minutes, although it took me 50 minutes on this occasion, which isn't too bad. It was 20c at 7pm the night before, yet here I was well wrapped up in my shorts and a woolly hat on a cold and sunny day stood on the esplanade and it was 7c. It felt like quite an achievement, which it was given that a few minutes of vacuuming would leave me aching and needing to sit down and rest a week earlier.

The final home straight as I strolled home was a struggle. The top of my right calf by my knee was really sore, and I was probably being overly optimistic in walking so far so soon. Nevertheless, I had to make an effort to get moving again.

My legs were aching, stiff and sore for days afterwards, which was predictable and I haven't been able to walk far or do much since. I was over the worst and the chronic fatigue and breathlessness had faded away, but I still faced a long haul to fully recover physically and mentally from what was a traumatic experience.

Life as we know it will never be the same again. I don't know what the long-term effects will be, and I am reluctant to travel abroad for the foreseeable future until some sort of normality returns. This virus doesn't recognise borders and it is impossible to do any sort of social-distancing on public transport or aircraft.

I can only focus on the present, knowing that I have been lucky and have made a swift recovery for the most part. This has been a life-changing experience and it crystallises your priorities.

Scientists and medical professionals are still learning about the virus, so diagnosing it and recovering from it is random and unpredictable.

I can't help but feel let down by the Scottish NHS prior to my hospital admission, as I had many of the tell-tale signs of COVID-19 yet it was dismissed as nothing more than a viral infection. The 111 system is not fit for purpose, and I do wonder how many lives have been lost as a result. I had to insist on being taken to hospital by ambulance and if I hadn't, I might not be here now to tell the tale.

Everyone's experience will be different and each will have their own story to tell. This is mine, and whilst I hope and expect to make a full recovery, I am left wondering if my immune system has been permanently damaged as a result. It's something I will have to manage and deal with on a risk-based approach, and I can't be complacent.

I can only take it one day at a time.

Connect with the Author

Want to stay in touch with Scott and be the first to hear about his new books?

Social media links:

Instagram: **@grumpy_g1t**

Twitter: **@grumpy_g1t**

Facebook: **The Complaints Resolver**

Websites: www.thegrumpygit.com

www.awriterinedinburgh.com

If you enjoyed this book, don't forget to leave a review on Amazon! I highly appreciate your reviews, and it only takes a minute to do.